PULL THE PLUG

ON OBAMACARE

A CITIZEN PAMPHLET

BY HOWARD HYDE

Copyright 2013 by Howard Hyde

Published by HHCapitalism.com

ISBN: 978-0615765938

Email: HHCapitalism@gmail.com

Twitter: @HowardHyde

TABLE OF CONTENTS

iv

Preface: It's Christmas Eve, 1776

In December 1776, the American revolutionary War for Independence was over, and the colonies had lost. Almost before the ink had dried on the Declaration of Independence of July 4 that year, the British general William Howe attacked New York, driving George Washington and the Continental Army into humiliating retreat. General Howe then pressed his advantage relentlessly through the fall. By December, it was all but finished. As the freezing temperatures and snow arrived, the confident British army demobilized for winter camp.

Further resistance by the rebels may have seemed pointless. Many Americans at that time may have thought that governance by a distant king was so prevalent on all other continents that there was no hope for independence from England.

But then the damndest thing happened: Washington didn't close shop for the winter like a gentleman, but on December 26 boldly launched a surprise attack on the British and Hessian mercenaries at Trenton, New Jersey, killing 21, wounding 90 and capturing 900, at a cost of four American wounded and not a single dead. The Revolution was not over after all. The United States of America might yet be more than a footnote to a forgotten rebellion.

Many Americans believe that the Patient Protection and Affordable Care Act, known variously as the P.P.A.C.A., the A.C.A. or Obamacare, is a done deal and something we just have to accept and learn to live with. Congress passed the law, the Supreme Court upheld it and Obama was re-elected along with a Democratic majority in the Senate. But a massively ambitious piece of legislation, based on mistaken premises, which can never fulfill its advertised promises and which is the crowning threat to the American constitutional civilization and economy since the American Revolution, cannot be surrendered to. The fact is, a growing majority of American citizens and legislators are already opposed to it. And as more and more supporters of Obamacare discover that they are personally among the millions whose access to affordable health care is being made *worse* by it, disenchantment will continue to grow.

This pamphlet is all about why we cannot concede defeat, why Obamacare must be rolled back, and what to replace it with. Whether you are a patient, a doctor, a legislator, a committed activist or just a middle-of-the-road guy or gal who can't understand what all the fuss is about, this plain-spoken, slightly irreverent citizen pamphlet will give you the intellectual ammunition necessary to understand America's predicament, defend your rights, and discuss solutions with your neighbors and your representatives.

We owe it to those Christmas 1776 patriots who gave us the incomparable gift that is the United States of America, and to future generations, who will read in the history books about us, our wisdom or our folly, our courage or our cowardice, as they either enjoy the estate we bequeath them, or struggle to pay the debts we put on their credit card.

Howard Hyde

February 2013

viii

Is this what you thought you were getting?

Nancy Pelosi, the Speaker of the House of Representatives who shepherded the Patient Protection and Affordable Care Act through her chamber in 2009 and 2010, once famously said that we need to pass the bill so that we can find out what's in it. Fair enough; now that it has passed, here's what's in it:

- Citizens who fail to enroll in a health insurance plan *approved by the Secretary of the Department of Health and Human Services* (HHS) will be **fined**: $285 in 2014; $975 in 2015; $2,085 in 2016. Your current plan may not qualify for approval, especially if it is a low-premium, high-deductible plan. See Section 1501 of the law.

- The IRS will withhold income tax refunds from taxpayers who fail to prove that they are enrolled in an HHS-approved plan.

- Employers of 50 or more full-time employees must provide an HHS-approved health plan or pay a fine of $2000 for each employee beyond the thirtieth. For example, an employer of 60 people would pay $2000 * 30 = $60,000. That's another employee or two who won't be getting hired.

- Insurance companies may not deny coverage or charge higher premiums to new applicants who are already sick and whose care is therefore almost guaranteed to cost more than the premiums the patient pays.

- Annual caps on insurance payouts are now illegal below $2 million, and will be illegal at any level in 2014.

- $716 billion will be siphoned out of Medicare to pay for Obamacare. Put another way, Obamacare is a makeover and massive expansion of Medicare; we're all Medicare patients now, or soon will be.

- Capital gains taxes (like the one that hits you when you sell your house after a lifetime of paying your mortgage on time) go up 3.8 percent on gains over $200,000.

- A 40% tax on high-end 'Cadillac' health care plans. If you like your plan, you can keep your plan, but only if you're willing and able to cough up thousands of dollars more, not in premiums or fees, but in tribute to Washington DC.

- No more low-premium, high-deductible plans allowed. Mini-Med plans such as the ones offered by McDonald's to entry-level workers, are now history.

- New limits on tax deductions for medical expenses. The threshold is now 10 percent of your income instead of 7.5 percent.

- The law creates the Independent Payment Advisory Board, or IPAB[1]. This will consist of 15 medical and economic 'experts' appointed by the president, employed exclusively by the government, with broad powers to rule on Medicare spending policy, including whether or not your life is worth the cost of preserving. Actually practicing private physicians are explicitly

[1] In earlier proposals of health care reform this was known by the name Independent Medicare Advisory Council (IMAC). The IPAB is created in Section 3405 of the Affordable Care Act.

consigned to the minority on the Board. The Board's organization and (lack of) accountability is modeled after the Federal Reserve Board. Its decisions may only be overruled by Congress with a 60 percent supermajority in the Senate.

- You will have to tell your boss how much money your spouse and children earn. Your employer is required by law to collect information about your *total household income* in order to classify you in the right 'affordability' category.

- Tax-free contributions to Flexible Spending Accounts or FSAs are capped at $2,500. Likewise, the use of Health Savings Accounts (HSAs) is restricted and deductibles are capped at $2,000 for individuals, $4,000 for families. These accounts may no longer be used to pay for over-the-counter drugs. Tax penalties for non-allowable purchases made through these accounts increase from 10 to 20 percent.

- Hospitals that spend the least dollars per senior patient get awarded bonus points by the government.

- The Medicare Part A payroll tax is hiked for taxpayers (like job-creating small business owners) who earn more than $200,000 individually or $250,000 as a couple.

- Funding for Medicare Advantage will be cut 27%. Each of its 7 million currently covered seniors will get on average $3,700 less allowance per year.

- The HHS now has authority over all physicians and their decisions, even if they are treating patients in private practice and/or under private insurance plans having nothing to do with Medicare or Medicaid.

- Spending to staff the government health care bureaucracy is expected to more than double to over $70 billion by the year 2020.

- Waivers: 1600 (and counting) special privileges of exemption from compliance with Obamacare's mandates have been awarded disproportionately to unions and groups that supported Obama's political agenda. Right, the waivers weren't written in the law, but they have become part of the policy implementation since the law passed. So finding out what's in it includes finding out that privileges, prejudices and enforcement will be arbitrary and based on political favoritism.

- People who don't get health coverage from their employer or from traditional government programs like Medicare and Medicaid are expected to shop for it at subsidized rates on 'exchanges' sponsored by the law, starting in 2014. The exchanges are marketplaces managed and policed by the HHS, and are where all of the above rules, regulations, standardization and mandates get put into practice. They are supposed to be set up by the states, but half of the states have so far refused to do the federal government's bidding, so presumably the federal government will set them up on its own in those states. Companies that offer health insurance to their employees will nevertheless be fined for failing to provide adequately if their employees opt for shopping on the exchanges.

- …and a whole lot of other stuff contained in its 2,500+ pages that none of the congressmen who voted on it read in its entirety.

Even though the law itself is comprised of over 2,500 pages of legalese, administrative departments like HHS still have the task of interpreting the law and writing the derived regulations that companies, individuals, patients and doctors are supposed to comply with. That will multiply the volume several times over.

Many of the nicest people you will ever meet supported the bill with the best of intentions, including most of this author's family and social circle. *But if every senator and representative in Congress – and the citizens who voted for them – had known that all of the above was in the bill, would it have passed?*

8

Obamacare misdiagnoses the problems

How did we get here again? Obamacare was variously sold to the public on the following premises:

- That there were 46 (casually rounded up to 50) million Americans without health insurance, and implicitly without access to care.

- That the U.S.A. lags behind other more enlightened countries that have universal health care, like Canada, the U.K. and France.

- That healthcare costs are out of control and getting worse, and a comprehensive reform led by Washington is the only solution.

- That private health insurance companies are greedy and/or evil parasites, or at least unsatisfactory.

- That free markets and free people can't provide optimum results in health care.

- That we must pass it in order to balance the budget.
- That we have to pass it so that we can find out what's in it.

None of these premises justify passage of the so-called Patient Protection and Affordable Care Act.

There are not 46 million victims

There are not now, nor have there ever been 46 million people in the United States without access to health care. As of 2009 there were:

- 10 million people earning $75,000 a year or more who did not purchase health insurance.
- 14 million people eligible for but not enrolled in government programs like the State Children's Health Insurance Program (S-CHIP), Medicaid and Medicare.
- 6 million people eligible for but not enrolled in health care plans from their private employer.

- Over 10 million immigrants, about half legal and half 'undocumented', without health insurance.
- A majority of Americans who were satisfied with their health insurance coverage.

In other words, over 25 million Americans chose of their own free will not to purchase health insurance even though they could afford it, and over 10 million people chose to come to this country even though health insurance was not automatically provided to them. Moreover, although some people are without insurance at some time during the year (such as when they are between jobs during a recession) that does not mean that they are unable to get insurance eventually; a minority are chronically uninsured.

These circumstances do not in any way constitute a crisis justifying massive new government intervention piled on top of 45 years of prior massive government intervention.

America needs to extend its lead, not catch up with anyone.

The U.S. health care system, for all its warts, is still the best that yet exists in the world. In 2000, the World Health Organization, applying the yardstick of government-controlled universal healthcare, ranked the U.S. system in 37th place in the world, based on that organization's judgment of 'financial fairness' and 'health distribution'. But nevertheless the WHO[2] was forced to concede that the U.S. is #1 in one minor area: actual patient care, or 'responsiveness to the needs of the patient'.

Life expectancy has advanced 50% in the U.S.A. in the last century to 73 years of age for men and 79 years for women. The average would be higher if not for our homicide, auto accident, obesity and tobacco smoking rates, which do not earn us laurels of national pride, but which have nothing to do with the quality and availability of health care. The relevant question to ask is, *what country do you want to be in when you are stabbed and bleeding in the street, involved in a traffic*

---

[2] Not to be confused with the British rock band of the same name.

collision or diagnosed with cancer? Your chances of survival and prospects for recovery are better here than anywhere else, whether you have insurance or not. Here are some facts and stats about health care <u>results</u> today:

Surviving Cancer:
- Breast cancer
  - U.S. survival rate: 90%
  - European survival rate: <80%
- Prostate cancer:
  - U.S. survival rate: 99%
  - Germany survival rate: 85%
  - Scotland survival rate: 71%
- Cancer in general (16 types):
  - U.S. men's 5-year survival rate: 66%
  - European men's 5-year survival rate: 47%
  - U.S. women's 5-year survival rate: 63%
  - European women's 5-year survival rate: 56%

More **Nobel prizes in Physiology or Medicine** are awarded to Americans than to researchers from any other country (many of these Americans are foreign-born doctors who found the freedom and opportunity to pursue their research here). Since 1950:

- U.S. Laureates: 81
- Rest of the world *combined*: 67

Considering that the U.S.A. holds only 5% of the world's population, that equates to scientists under our system being *23 times more effective* in achieving breakthrough research than those working under other economic and political systems.

Likewise, 80% of medical innovation worldwide comes from the U.S.A.

More stats:

- Cardiac disease death rates have fallen over 60% in 50 years.

- Polio is virtually history in the U.S.A.

- Childhood leukemia is now a treatable disease, whereas it once killed almost every child that it touched.

- AIDS or HIV-positive immunodeficiency is now a chronic disease instead of being the death sentence that it was in the 1980's.

A survey conducted jointly by the Kaiser Family Foundation, ABC News and USA Today, released in October 2006, found that 89 percent of Americans were satisfied with their own personal medical care. 93% of insured Americans who had recently suffered a serious illness were satisfied with their health care. So were 95% of those who suffered from chronic illness. 70 percent of the uninsured who indicated their level of satisfaction said they were either "satisfied" or "very satisfied" with their health care, and only 17.5 percent said they were "very dissatisfied". 64% of American women said they would rather have a private than government plan.

By comparison, here are some features of health care systems in other parts of the world that Obamacare intends to emulate in order that we should 'catch up':

- In Britain, the government-sponsored National Institute for Health and Clinical Excellence (NICE) determines whether a drug's development will be funded. Not pharmaceutical companies, not private investors, not non-profit charitable foundations.

16

- The same NICE people decide whether a seriously ill patient will receive an expensive treatment that could save or prolong his/her life. This is real Rationing by Committee, a.k.a. the 'death panels' that Sarah Palin was excoriated for suggesting was a part of Obamacare. The Independent Payment Advisory Board (IPAB) is the American version of this committee, created by the new law.

- A patient in Britain undergoing major surgery faces a risk of death four times higher than a similar patient in the U.S.; a patient that is seriously ill in Britain is seven times more likely to die than one in the U.S..

- Canada has a 'single-payer' system. Only the government pays directly for health care costs, and doctors are *prohibited* from seeing patients privately on a cash basis; the private practice of medicine has been explicitly abolished. The result? The Canadian system is characterized by long waiting lists for urgent treatment, referrals, MRIs and life-saving care. Here are some Canadian stats:

Copyright 2013 by Howard Hyde. All rights reserved.
www.HHCapitalism.com

- 41 days average wait for an MRI in Alberta.

- 10 percent of knee-replacement patients wait more than 616 days in Saskatchewan.

- 201 days average wait for hip replacement surgery in Nova Scotia (that's *after* obtaining the referral from the family doctor. BUT…)

- 15% of Canadians can't find a family doctor to refer them for MRIs, knee or hip replacements or anything else, due to a doctor shortage.

- The U.S.A. has four times as many MRI machines per capita than Canada has. It is easier to get an MRI for a dog or cat or even a horse than for a human being in Canada; the government doesn't ration and regulate veterinary care to the degree it does for homo sapiens patients.

- Canadians receive less preventive care than Americans. Cannucks are 20% less likely than Yankees to have a colonoscopy; 30% less likely to have a PSA test; 10% less likely to have a Pap smear; 15% less likely to have a mammogram.

Overall, the average wait for specialized care in Canada is 18 weeks. For orthopedic surgery, like knee and hip replacements that enable you to walk again, the national average wait is 40 weeks. That's 9 months. Average. It wasn't always like this; wait times have worsened by 91 percent over 19 years.

In short, Canada's health care system is hailed as 'fairer' than the U.S. by Michael Moore and others, yet the only thing fair about it is that everyone is more equally miserable in Canada.

Is this the system we want to emulate in the U.S.A? Do we honestly imagine that *our* politicians and bureaucrats are smarter, more competent and less corrupt than their Canadian counterparts, and therefore we will be immune to these inevitable consequences of government command and control? Canadians who don't want to wait 18 weeks and are able, cross the border into the U.S. and pay cash to get care. Where will they go when the U.S. system is no better than the Canadian one? Where the millions of other willing-to-pay foreigners go?

In the freest and most prosperous nation in the history of the world, there has never been greater quality care nor greater access to it by the most common of citizens, you and me.

Out of Control Costs?

"The explosion in health-care costs has put our federal budget on a disastrous path."

Barack Obama, March 2009

Almost everyone is concerned about the cost of health care rising faster than inflation. Even so, prior to the passage of the A.C.A., health care expenditures in the U.S.A. had been growing at their lowest rate in 40 years. In 1970, the growth rate was 10.5%; in 1980, 13%; in 1990, 11%. In 2007, 2008 and 2009 the numbers were, respectively: 6.1%, 4.7% and 3.8%. Health care cost inflation was declining, not exploding, not in crisis.

And even if it were a crisis, the automatic conclusion that only the government can set things right is without foundation. The evidence suggests the

20

opposite. Now that the law has passed, the actuaries of the HHS, the primary agency responsible for rule-making, implementation and enforcement for Obamacare, are projecting that costs will rise by 7.8% in 2014, with 30% of that being the federal share. Health entitlement spending is rising to 24% of the federal budget in 2013 from 21% in 2012. The Congressional Budget Office (CBO) estimates that federal health spending will account for over 10% of the entire economy in the next generation, up from 5.4% today. Is this the solution to out-of-control health care costs?

What ~~cockroaches~~ insurance companies?

A neutral unbiased objective moderator at an Obamacare debate at a medical school once quipped that "insurance companies are like cockroaches", echoing the sentiments of many Americans. Fair enough; we're all familiar with serious scholarly expositions such as the *Insuricare* scene in the Pixar animated movie *The Incredibles* and we nodded our heads in recognition of the corruption and greed. But the fact of the matter is that medical insurance companies such as we know them today are not insurance companies at all in the true meaning of that term. Rather they are Frankenstein-monster products of the prior rounds of political mandates and prohibitions and their inevitable consequences, corruption and lack of concern for the well-being of their supposed clients. At best they function increasingly like micro-managed public utilities. Would you buy a health plan from your gas and water company? In effect, you probably already have.

Most of us buy (real) insurance for things other than health care because we don't want to be financially wiped out if something rare but catastrophic happens. We buy automobile, homeowner's, boat, renter's, fire, earthquake and flood insurance just in case something terrible, unwanted and unlikely happens. It is true that some automobile companies offer pre-paid plans for oil changes and routine maintenance, but that is not insurance. Moreover, just because we buy auto insurance doesn't mean we can have any car we want; we are still limited to Hyundai's or Ferraris depending

22

on our wealth, tastes and choices. We buy at the intersection of our needs and our means. We insure against eventualities that we cannot afford.

What we call 'health insurance' today is hardly that at all. Instead it increasingly takes the form of a pre-paid maintenance plan as 'managed care', Health Maintenance Organizations (HMOs) and/or Accountable Care Organizations (ACOs), in which the government or a government-regulated corporation – not the consumer/patient or the insurer – decides the terms and features of the contract. Government regulation of the health insurance market has suppressed the 'insurance' part in favor of pre-paid maintenance with teaser goodies like contraception, hair plugs, fertility treatments, sports club memberships and massage therapy. These are not the 'terrible, unwanted and unlikely' things that insurance was invented for. Coverage for catastrophic injuries, illness and hospitalization – the original legitimate purpose of health insurance – has almost become an afterthought.

Free Markets don't work... except where they are tried.

The argument that free markets cannot solve the problems of health care is a willful denial of the overwhelming evidence that free markets are precisely what deliver the greatest wealth of goods and services at the lowest possible prices to the greatest number of people.

In every market where private enterprise, private property rights and voluntary cooperation prevail, prices relative to wages have steadily fallen year after year, decade after decade and generation after generation, while quality has improved and innovation has flourished. That is how the U.S.A. came to be the most prosperous nation ever on Earth; by being the least restrictive of citizen's freedom and most supportive of private property rights.

Only ten years ago "I phone" was a banal subject-verb expression. Now those syllables identify one of the most miraculous products ever brought to market at a price affordable to hundreds of millions of ordinary people around the world, in spite of having

24

more computer processing power and totally cool features per unit than the entire NASA Apollo program that put American astronauts on the moon a generation ago. Captain Kirk of the Starship Enterprise, two hundred years in the future, hardly had (will have?) that much power in the Communicator gadget into which he commanded 'Beam us up, Scotty!'

In contrast, wherever markets are dominated by government regulation or outright monopoly, the norm is to find deteriorating quality of products and services, shortages, waiting lists, rationing, inflation, poor customer/citizen service and a host of other ills. There's a reason that jumbo jet airplanes, web browsers, flat-screen TVs and smart phones were invented in capitalist countries and not in, say, Hugo Chavez's Venezuela. Advocates for socialized economies need to spend more time in such countries – living as the common citizens do, not as trendy tourists.

When governments get out of the way, private innovation thrives. The Safeway supermarket company successfully beat its own healthcare cost inflation while simultaneously improving the health of its workforce through its Healthy Measures program, on its own initiative.

The problems of America's health care system are not the product of a free market. On the contrary, medicine is the most highly controlled sector of our economy (OK, nuclear bomb manufacture may be slightly more regulated, but that may be justified given the slightly more elite clientele). And the government throws its weight around to influence market behavior through hundreds of federal and state agencies, spending a million times millions of dollars (that's what trillions are in case you hadn't thought it through: millions of millions[3]).

We will have more to say about the economics of markets in medical products and services in later chapters.

---

[3] To get an idea of how big a trillion is, think of something very small, like a second in time. A trillion seconds is approximately 35,000 years. A string of one trillion Ping-Pong balls could be wrapped around Planet Earth one thousand times.

New Budget-Balancing Technique: Massive Expansion of Entitlement Programs

To quote Barack Obama: "It will reduce our deficit by over $100 billion over the next decade and more than $1 trillion the decade after that".

Will those who believe that creating a massive new government entitlement program targeting 50 million citizens will actually help the government spend less money, please raise your hand? The only justification for such a belief is that politicians and bureaucrats will be far more competent in managing this sector of the economy from the top down than the patients, physicians, employers and insurance companies that nominally manage it now. Where is the evidence of past governmental success to substantiate such a claim?

The idea becomes all the more absurd when we learn that the principal source of funding for Obamacare is our largest unfunded, bankrupt entitlement program: Medicare. Read on.

28

It harms more than it solves

The so-called Affordable Care Act:

- Cannibalizes existing insolvent programs.

- Violates the sacred trust among patients, caregivers and families.

- Steam-rolls over the traditional model of the independent, self-employed (small business) practice of medicine. It accelerates the trend of herding physicians into employee roles in large hospital corporations and managed-care organizations (MCOs), or putting them out of business altogether.

- Redefines the constitutional relationship between the federal government and the states.

- Fundamentally alters the relationship between the American citizen and the state.

- Reduces the availability and affordability of medical services (no matter what the law's name says).

30

Medical Care Supply and Demand, Art and Science

It offends the refined sensibilities of many high-minded people that the free market, that vulgar 'law of the jungle', should have any place in the sacred and transcendent fields of health, education, the arts and so on. But just as the laws of chemistry certainly apply to drugs and their effect on the body, likewise there is no rational reason to expect that economic laws shouldn't apply to the production and distribution of health care products and services. If more people are clamoring for services that fewer people are providing, it is inevitable that either the price of that service will go up or the availability will go down, and the consequence will be shortages, queues, waiting lists, black markets and other forms of de facto rationing.

That's the law of Supply and Demand, and it's real, it is of the fundamental nature of human action in society, and like the law of gravity, it is not subject to repeal via political legislation.

The practice of medicine involves a whole lot of math and science (something which our public school

Copyright 2013 by Howard Hyde. All rights reserved.
www.HHCapitalism.com

pupils and public government politicians are woefully deficient in) but at its core it is and of necessity must be an *art*: an art of scientific inquiry and social interaction among doctor, family and patient; the whole patient, not just the pancreas; the patient's family history, not just today's symptoms; the patient's personality type, temperament, psychological profile, intimate and casual relationships, work, nutrition, exercise, sleep and drug habits, not just ink bubbles on a computer chart. Just as a musician must practice scales, rehearse repertoire and participate in concerts, physicians must study, practice and perform for years to develop their knowledge, polish their technique and perfect the personal *style* that suits them and their patients the best. It is no accident that in Greek mythology, Apollo was the god of both music and medicine[4].

---

[4] For a fascinating exposition of the arguments among allopathic, chiropractic, homeopathic, naturopathic and osteopathic physicians, see <u>Divided Legacy</u> by Harris Coulter. It's not that one branch of medicine is scientific and the other is not; it's that science is a never-ending quest for understanding and truth, which can't be legislated or bottled in bureaucratic codes.

32

Yet the government-sanctioned system for regulating healthcare services completely undermines the very essence of medical practice – the physician's art. In the sterile bureaucratic calculus, a bypass operation is a bypass operation is a bypass operation, whether performed by a rookie resident or a world-renowned surgeon with 30 years of experience. Every act of the physician has been digitized to a payment code (known as the Common Procedural Technology or CPT code) in the computer system with a value set by Medicare which administrators will reimburse, no more, no less, with no qualifiers, no accounting for skill, experience, dexterity or judgment, no allowance or toleration for individualized care; no exceptions.

If all there were to medicine was the correct generic, commodity cookie-cutter treatment for the matching generic disease or condition, then no physicians with 12 years of post-secondary education and training would be required; only kindergarten-variety desk monkeys instructed on how to put the square pegs into the square holes would be necessary.

A physician who treats a patient according to his or her professional judgment differently from what the government-sanctioned 'evidence-based' protocol[5] says he or she should do faces the risk of denial of reimbursement, second-guessing of his/her decision, loss of license or worse. It is happening today with Medicare billings and pharmaceutical prescriptions, and it will explode tenfold when the Medicare model is applied to the entire population.

"Doctors are bound by federal law to follow protocols set forth in Washington DC. Deviation can be punished, and how they are going to punish is hard to figure out. My reputation now is based on taking good care of patients. In the future my reputation is going to be whether I stick to protocols."

-Dr. Jeffrey English, Neurologist, Atlanta GA

Under Obamacare, the Independent Payment Advisory Board (IPAB) may deny Medicare patients medicine, devices or treatments that its 'comparative effectiveness analysis' algorithm deems unsatisfactory, meaning too costly it's about the cost to the agency,

---

[5] produced by the 'embedded clinical decision support' – the computer that tells the doctor what to do.

not the effectiveness to the patient). The most personal service that exists is directed by the most impersonal agency at 3,000 miles' distance. And that most impersonal of all agencies now owns your very life.

Meanwhile, doctors who are able to are moving into elite concierge practices catering to VIPs (the 0.0001%) or selling out their businesses to accountable care organizations (ACOs). The overhead cost in money, time, information technology, data collection, and reporting required to comply with the law and related regulations means that only the biggest fish (and corporations) can survive. Historically the majority of doctors in the U.S. have been in private practice. By 2014, two thirds of them will be employees of increasingly large corporations. The top doctors will not be seeing you and me; they will be busy flipping medical practice businesses to bigger buyers, like internet startup companies in the late 1990s. Nice boom if you can get it.

Cannibalizing Medicare

How do you suppose Obamacare covers its (lowball estimate) $1,000,000,000,000 ten-year price tag? In part by taking $716,000,000,000 away from the Medicare program. Medicare was enacted by the federal government in 1965 to provide universal coverage for the elderly, of whom by the way we're getting a lot more as the post-World War II 'baby boom' generation cruises past 65. Before Obamacare arrived, the program was already insolvent, heading for bankruptcy before the end of this decade. You can't finance a new entitlement this way any more than you can save a boat from sinking by pumping water out of the bow and pouring it into the stern.

"Cuts to Medicare from 2013 through 2022 will total $716 billion. These are comprised of a $269 billion cut to hospital services, $156 billion in cuts to Medicare Advantage programs, $145 billion to DHS payments and other Medicare provisions, $66 billion to home health services, $39 billion in cuts to 'other services', and $17 billion to hospice services."

-Adam Dorin, MD, America's Medical Society

So what problems have been solved by looting Medicare?

Perhaps the math will come out fine in the end because the government will eliminate 'waste, fraud and abuse', which is widely acknowledged to be rampant in Medicare and other government programs. But where is the evidence that an even bigger, more universal system of healthcare, covering not just seniors but 100% of the population from cradle to grave, will be any less prone to waste, fraud and abuse than a much smaller program?

How will the administrators of Medicare handle any shortfall? Among other things, they will reduce reimbursements to doctors for services rendered to patients. But this will only exacerbate problems that already exist with this program. Doctors are already opting out of Medicare and Medicaid contracts as fast as they can because it's a money-losing proposition for them. The threat of a 27% cut in Medicare reimbursements to doctors has been postponed (again) as of January 2013, but it still hasn't been eliminated.

"My group left Medicaid about six or seven years ago because we could not care for patients adequately so we felt uncomfortable in the system and the reimbursement was such that it was actually costing us more to see the patients – being a Medicaid provider – *than if we just didn't take them and saw them for free should they be in the hospital*" [author's emphasis]

-Dr. Jeffrey English, Neurologist, Atlanta GA

Obama's promise that "if you like your doctor, you can keep your doctor" may (or not) hold technically true in terms of the letter of the law, but if the actual effect of the law is to drive doctors out of practice, you won't be able to keep the one you like. The fact is that today more than 80% of American physicians are contemplating retiring early, quitting medicine or at least decreasing office hours.

States become Administrative Departments of the Federal Government

Under the U.S. Constitution the States are independent sovereign entities that surrender to the Federal government only the functions that are common to all the states collectively, like national defense, diplomacy and trade with other nations. But under Obamacare, states are treated as if they were mere administrative departments tasked with carrying out orders (such as to set up health insurance exchanges) from Washington. France's government is explicitly structured this way. So what's wrong with the French model? We're not here to criticize the wine or the cheese; especially the latter puts our own to shame[6]. But among the poorest states in the western hemisphere are those whose legal and economic legacy comes to us courtesy of Napoleon Bonaparte; think Louisiana, Quebec and Haiti. France does not provide a viable economic model for America to follow. There is a reason our Constitution defines the relationship of the federal government to

---

[6] The author lived in France for 4 years.

the states the way that it does, differently from European parliamentary systems. If the Constitution is deemed unsatisfactory, there are provisions for its amendment. That's not something to be undertaken casually, nor by stealth.

Are you a Citizen...or a Subject?

Starting in 2014, you will be required to enroll in a health care plan, not necessarily one of your choosing, but one which is approved by the federal government. Read this warm-and-fuzzy legalese: "SEC. 1311(h)(I). Beginning on January 1, 2015, a qualified health plan may contract with…(B) a health care provider only if such provider implements such mechanisms to improve health care quality as the Secretary may by regulation require."

You must prove that you are enrolled in such a plan on your income tax statement. Under the Obamacare law, the IRS has budgeted for 16,000 additional agents in order to enforce compliance. Expect audits to increase.

Furthermore, your personal electronic medical record (EMR) will become the property of the state. Next time you are handed a HIPPA[7] 'privacy notice' at a medical facility, read the fine print. In some places people have noticed under the heading of 'National Security' a statement to the effect that the treating medical facility may disclose your health information to federal officials "in order to protect the President, other officials or foreign heads of state."

Privacy is growing harder to come by. That embarrassing infection you got in college? Should have gone to Cuba to get it treated; it is now accessible to the government. Those antidepressants you went on after your cat died? Should have procured them on the black market. "Please confirm how many plastic surgeries you have had, Madam [your name here _____] candidate for job/position/office?" Remember when your third grade teacher caught you tinkling behind the bungalow, sent you to the principal's office and told you "this is going on your permanent record"? Now they really mean it.

---

[7] Health Insurance Portability and Accountability Act

Does the right to privacy have any value to the supporters of Obamacare? Just asking.

As it so often goes with many 'technology-will-solve-all-of-our-problems' promises, EMRs are turning out to be not quite the panacea they were sold to be[8]. Navigating the menus and filling out the fields of an EMR app is a time-consuming and frustrating process for many doctors and their staff which takes time and attention away from the actual flesh-and-blood human being patient sitting in the exam room. If the next time you visit your doctor he or she doesn't seem to be looking at or listening to you as attentively as before, but seems preoccupied with some computer gadget, you'll know why.

EMRs may be a good idea that fulfill their promise eventually. But brute-force government mandates are not the way to get there.

[8] For the record, the author is an IT Specialist.

43

It won't accomplish what its supporters claim

Here is a sampling of what the White House and/or various promoters of the bill claim it would achieve:

- More affordable coverage – bring down the cost of health care.

- Better access to care.

- Stronger Medicare.

- Stronger consumer rights and protections.

- No disruption to existing satisfactory policies and services. "If you're one of the more than 250 million Americans who already have health insurance, you will keep your insurance." - Barack Obama

- Reduce health insurance premiums for the average family by $2,500 per year.

- Cuts to the national deficit by over two hundred billion dollars during its first 10 years; cut it by over a Trillion dollars over the next two decades.

- Universal coverage; health insurance and care for every American citizen regardless of ability to pay.
- All preventative care free on all insurance plans.
- Guaranteed coverage for children of primary insureds up to age 26.
- Reward doctors for quality over quantity.

It Already Isn't Working.

Premiums are rising, and are expected to go up 50% on average, with the historically low-cost states seeing the greatest increase. In some markets they will double. The mandates to cover everyone regardless of age or preexisting condition with a bundle of benefits dictated by Washington and with controls on price differentiation are all driving the costs up, as they must.

Small businesses are getting hit especially hard. The employer mandate will increase the cost of hiring by $1.79 per hour or more per employee on average. It gives employers incentives to drop coverage, slow hiring, increase layoffs and/or replace low-wage workers with part-timers, offshore/foreign contractors or machines.

As of January 2013, premiums for families are $5,500 more expensive on average than Obama promised they would be (he said they would go down $2,500; instead they are up $3,000). Now that the law has passed, premiums increased 9% in 2011-2012 and are expected by the actuaries at the HHS itself to rise by 7.8% in 2014, compared to a 5% prior annual rate of increase. Health entitlement spending is rising to 24% of the federal budget in 2013, up from 21% in 2012. The Congressional Budget Office (CBO) estimates that federal government health spending will account for over 10% of the entire economy in the next generation, up from 5.4% today. This is the solution to out-of-control health care costs? This will bring down the deficit?

"Because we say so"

A random walk among websites and other sources that support Obamacare reveals that in large part they consider the law a success not because of its actual outcomes, but because of what it 'does'. For example, the law orders all insurers to cover dependent

46

children up to the age of 26, then claims credit for providing the benefit to millions of 'children' at the stroke of a pen. But ordering people to do something and achieving the outcome that you profess are not the same thing. Passing the law does nothing to actually produce the $3,000 per year additional wealth required on average to cover these 'children'. Some organizations will not be able to afford it. One of the earliest casualties of this mandate was, of all people, the union SEIU United Healthcare Workers of New York, which had previously been covering about 6,000 dependent children of its members up to the age of 23. The mandate to cover dependent children to 26 years was a contributing factor to pushing this union over its own fiscal cliff, compelling it to drop the plan for the 6,000 children of its 30,000 members. Large, well-endowed universities like Harvard and Yale may be able to continue providing health insurance plans for students. But smaller colleges are already feeling the squeeze from the new law. Lenoir-Rhyne University of Hickory, North Carolina, the University of Puget Sound in Tacoma, Washington and Cornell College of Mount Vernon, Iowa are among the institutions of higher learning that can no longer afford to offer student health insurance plans. Expect to hear more announcements of companies, universities and other organizations dropping their coverage.

Likewise mandating 'free' preventive care to the insured does not make it free to provide. As the Nobel laureate in economics Milton Friedman famously said, there's no such thing as a free lunch; someone has to pay for it. Insurance companies will have to raise fees and/or limit coverage on other parts of their policies in order to recompense their costs of offering 'free' preventive care.

The rationale behind free preventive care is that it will lead to savings down the road by avoiding the need to care for more serious, un-prevented illness. That's a reasonable theory, and insurance companies should certainly be free to package their offerings in such a way that limits their own risk of exposure to higher claim expenses. They have every incentive to do so. But mandating a one-size-fits-all solution from Washington does not permit the market to function in finding the optimum plan for each individual patient.

And so it will go with every mandate, micromanagement and overregulation. Unintended (and sometime intended but unspoken) consequences will drive some institutions out of the business of providing health insurance if not out of business altogether. People who have private coverage will lose it. People who are satisfied with the quality of their care will see that quality deteriorate. Doctors will be rewarded for compliance with protocols that require less education and expertise to follow, but they may be fined, stiffed or de-licensed for exercising their own independent professional judgment.

A History of Cost Overruns.

The U.S. Medicare system, when proposed in 1965, was expected to cost $12 billion by 1990; It actually cost $90 billion in that year - seven and a half times more than the public had been led to expect. Is Obamacare going to be any different?

Similarly, Medicaid was projected to cost $238 million per year. In its first year alone, the actual invoice came in at $1 billion - almost four times greater than advertised. The hospitalization program was supposed to cost $1 billion by 1987; instead the tab was $17 billion that year. The program has been expanded to the point of being 37 times more costly (inflation-adjusted) than originally sold.

Yet we are supposed to believe that we have a unfettered free market in health care ruled only by the law of the jungle and that it is insufficient regulation that is causing all of the problems, and that the only rational solution now is for the federal government, with its stellar track record, to take command of a sixth or more of the entire U.S. economy.

How well have other countries that provide universal coverage managed their healthcare costs?

The Canadian health care system's unfunded liability as of 2010 was 537,700,000,000 Canadian dollars; over half a trillion. That's a third of the entire country's GDP, or $33,000 per every Canadian taxpayer.

50

Politicians need to credibly explain why the U.S.A. should be immune to such problems before committing to such a massive program.

Why it must and will certainly fail

Obamacare, the most ambitious social entitlement program ever attempted in the U.S., will only magnify and multiply the failures of prior interventions.

The failures of Medicare, Medicaid and socialized health care systems around the world are not accidents, nor rounding errors, nor even the unfortunate results of incompetent management and staff. Rather, they are the inevitable, predictable result of forceful interference in the voluntary cooperation of free citizens. Obamacare will fail for the same reason that the Soviet Union failed: command-and-control economies cannot function rationally.

When President Ronald Reagan famously declared "Mr. Gorbachev, tear down this wall" in 1987, few people believed that the concrete and razor-wire barrier separating the communist East from the free West Berlin, Germany, would in fact be demolished just 2 years later, liberating the citizen-inmates not only of the eastern sector of Berlin but of most of Eastern Europe and the Soviet Union itself. But Reagan understood that any system that denied individual liberty as both the fundamental moral principle of civilization and as the only rational basis for functioning economics, was doomed to collapse under its own weight. He understood this in part because the inevitable downfall of the Soviet system had been predicted a few years earlier…in 1922.

Ludwig von Mises, the Austrian-American economist, demonstrated that Socialism could never fulfill its promise no matter what variation was attempted nor how wise and virtuous the men running it. In his book *Socialism,* Mises clearly demonstrated that every wage and price control, every tariff, tax, privilege, prejudice, manipulation and regulation that does not derive from government's legitimate need to prevent and punish murder, robbery, assault, fraud, theft, rape, persecution and conspiracy – every such interference distorts and destroys *information* necessary for rational economic planning and action on the part of individuals. If some collective entity like the state owns or otherwise controls capital goods, land, natural resources, factories, machinery, services, etc. then there is

- **no market** for these goods
- no **buying and selling,**
- no **bargaining and haggling,**
- no **competition** to compel **lower prices, higher quality, better service** and the **division of labor** where each finds the role they are best suited to.
- no dynamic play of the law of **Supply and Demand.**

If there is no market then there are **no prices** in the real sense of the word. Prices constitute the **indispensable information system** for signaling the needs and scarcities in an economy, and the cost of available alternatives. There are a hundred different ways to build a building, and dozens of alternative materials and techniques for each component. Which combination is the most economical? Who knows? Without prices, there is no way of knowing. There is no other metric that can adequately substitute for market prices. Economic planning cannot function without these numbers.

That is why Socialism fails every time it is tried: **Economic calculation is impossible under Socialism**.

And then there's the (see Mises' book with the same title) *Bureaucracy*. Without markets there is no competition, neither incentive nor reward for better customer service or for providing a higher quality product at a lower price. The entire economy ends up being managed like a giant post office or department of motor vehicles, bleeding taxpayer money and staffed by government workers insulated by iron-clad privileges, job security and pensions that do not vary with how well or how poorly they serve willing (or unwilling) customers. It is not that the people who work for such institutions are bad people; to the contrary. The problem is that the systems of incentives, constraints, accountability and reward under which they labor are not responsive to the needs of the people they are supposed to serve.

As applied to the health care market, these same principles apply. The more the government commands and controls services, insurance, physicians and other health professionals, drugs/pharmaceuticals, equipment like MRI machines and devices like defibrillators etc. then the result is

- **a less flexible and innovative market** for these,
- **less buying and selling** between parties commanding their own resources on their own account and for their own benefit or risk,
- **less bargaining and haggling** (apart from government bullying from its position of monopoly power, as in price controls shrinking Medicare payment schedules etc.),
- **less open competition** to compel **lower prices, higher quality, better service** and the **division of labor**
- **less** functioning of **Supply and Demand**.

The inevitable consequences will be:
- the suppression of **Profit and Loss** as legitimate regulators of behavior or scorecards of success or failure,

- a reduced scope of the operation of **Prices**, leading to a breakdown of the indispensible economic **information system** of abundance, scarcity and alternatives,

- **fewer medical and pharmaceutical innovations** due to the reduced possibility of recovering the costs of research and development; why bet billions when success makes you a political target?

- **shortages, waiting lists** and government-imposed **rationing** of dwindling services, doctors and medicinal drugs.

With the suppression of a rational, market-based economy, what emerges is bureaucratic management directed by politically-derived values. The opinions, concerns and desires of physicians, patients and families take a back seat to functionaries who are removed from personal economic or emotional involvement or ethical responsibility in the patient's case. What matters to the bureaucrat is that he faithfully execute the rules dictated to him by the dominant political party, legalistic sub-paragraphs

56

buried inside 10,000-page tomes like the federal register, and union bosses.

'Progressive' politicians often feed on the consumer's resentment of 'faceless' bureaucrats at private insurance companies, and attribute the evils that these companies commit to the failure of the free market. But when we reach the point where there is only one insurance company left standing, the government, with the right to tax you, fine you or deny you services rather than take losses on its own account, people aren't going to love that 'insurance company' more than the few nominally private ones they have now. Even if private insurance companies survive Obamacare, they will be taking their orders from the government regulators and the unelected and unaccountable czars; not from you and me the patients, families and physicians; not from the free market.

Supporters of Obamacare deny that it is socialism on the grounds that the law neither nationalizes the insurance companies nor provides a 'public option' from the Federal government (*yet* – give it time). But if private citizens from patients to physicians to insurance companies are no longer free to do as they see fit with what is theirs and to exchange (or not) freely with whom they wish on mutually agreeable terms as long as no criminal activity is involved, then by definition we have arrived at a form of socialism. The National Socialist Worker's Party in Germany in the 1930's and 40's (affectionately known as the Nazis) did not nationalize all industry in Germany; they just gave orders on what to produce, in what quantity, and what to sell to whom at what prices: command-and-control. Otherwise business firms were left nominally under private ownership. It was not private capitalist entrepreneurs who came up with the idea of invading all the neighbors and gassing Jews, gypsies and 'undesirables'. Rather, anyone who fell under Hitler's power was ordered on pain of labor camps and/or death to comply with His orders. It is the general infringement upon liberty and private property rights on the part of government that constitute socialism, not the specific form that that infringement takes. By virtue of the government telling us what we may and may not do to a degree unprecedented in American history, the A.C.A. fits the definition of socialized medicine. President Obama is not Hitler (neither is George W. Bush, even if some disagree). But his ambition for commanding and controlling the American economy and the liberty of American citizens differs with the more virulent forms of socialism only by degree.

We began this pamphlet by recapping the justifications for Obamacare, including the idea that we must do something about the 46 million uninsured, which turns out to be a completely misleading number. But according to a Congressional Budget Office (CBO) study, 30 million Americans are *still* projected to be without health insurance in the year 2022, in spite of everything that Obamacare does. It won't accomplish its core objective.

Socialized medicine is not a new idea. It has been tried again and again in many advanced countries yet it has never achieved results to compare with the relatively free United States. Obamacare, the biggest such initiative of them all, is destined to be the biggest failure of them all. The most sincere and well-meaning supporters of the Patient Protection and Affordable Care Act may very well end up becoming the most disappointed.

So what do we replace it with?

What should we do instead of Obamacare? Since almost everything about it goes 180 degrees in the wrong direction, for the most part we can start by taking its opposite. For example:

✓ Allow consumers, providers and insurers to negotiate coverage, benefits and prices without interference. Let a thousand flowers bloom, rather than dictating to insurance companies what their plans must and may not cover, as Obamacare does.

✓ Increase rather than reduce the number of medical products that taxpayers are allowed to cover using flexible spending accounts (FSAs) and health savings accounts (HSAs), and increase the level of permissible contributions to the same.

✓ Cancel all new taxes, government fees and penalties created by the law. This includes:

- The Individual Mandate, a.k.a. the 'it's-not-called-a-tax-in-the-bill-and-the-promoters-denied-it-was-a-tax-but-it-IS-a-tax-for-convenience-of-constitutional-review-purposes' tax.
- The Hospital Insurance portion of the payroll tax, (up 31% as of January 2013).
- The Obamacare surcharge of 0.9% on the payroll tax.
- The medical device tax. We need more medical devices at lower prices, not fewer at higher.
- The tax on medical drugs. We need more of them at lower prices, not fewer at higher.

Cancelling these taxes will allow economic growth, investment and dynamic innovation to deliver the services, products, choices, lower prices and higher tax revenue that benefit all citizens, the taxpayers and government at all levels. The alternative is micromanaging a stagnating, shrinking economy. If you believe the taxes don't affect you because you're not 'rich', think again; high taxes get passed along to you in the form of higher prices and more limited choices.

- ✓ Make all health care plans tax exempt. When the government taxes something, it creates incentives to produce less of that thing. Wasn't the idea to get *more* people on to health care plans? Obamacare taxes 'Cadillac' healthcare plans at 40%, so instead of costing $20,000 or more, they will cost $28,000 or more.

  Today's luxury goods are tomorrow's Wal-Mart commodities. Just as personal computers, cell phones, automatic transmission and air bag crash safety systems were once luxuries that only the rich could afford, under the natural progress of free markets the features of so-called 'Cadillac plans' will become increasingly affordable to all.

- ✓ Expand the tax deductibility of medical expenses by setting the floor at zero percent instead of raising it from 7.5 to 10 percent. Shouldn't an act of Congress entitled 'Affordable Care' make medical expenses more affordable?

- ✓ Increase tax deductions and/or credits for expenses on medical services, products and

64

devices. It may 'cost' the government money, but the money will be more wisely and effectively spent when it is in the hands of the citizen.

✓ Index tax thresholds for inflation. At the rate things are going, faster than we know it, $250,000 will be the new poverty line, with the tax rates conceived for 'the rich'.

✓ Eliminate the mandate on the use of Electronic Medical Records (EMRs) and allow patients, providers and insurers to work out whatever arrangement emerges from voluntary cooperation in a free market. Patients in particular should have the option (enforceable by law and security) of owning their own EMR in the same way that they own and manage their own checking, saving, credit and investment accounts online. It's property of the most private kind.

✓ Just Say No to the law's 'exchanges' scheme. The insurance exchanges created by the law are not markets; Sally Pipes aptly calls them 'regulatory corrals'. They exist to facilitate micromanagement of medical plans and services, features and prices, telling everyone what to do and how to do it.

They are the command-and-control cells of the federal government's long arm.

The 'Replace' part of 'Repeal and Replace' would be well-guided by the following principles:

Legalize real *health insurance ...across the fruited plain*

The vast majority of the laws regulating health insurance plans – from required benefits to covered conditions to eligibility and permissible premiums – should be repealed, leaving these aspects to the voluntary cooperation of the market. If people want to buy pre-paid oil change and maintenance plans and companies wish to provide them, they should be at liberty to do so. If people just want coverage for catastrophic illnesses or accidents and nothing else, the market will price that plan (low premium, high deductible). Not every insurance company will offer every option to every person in every market, any more than Starbucks, Wal-Mart or Bloomingdale's do. But more freedom will lead to more options and choices all around, resulting in more people getting the coverage that suits them best (not the coverage that suits the Secretary of the Department of H.H.S. best).

Legalizing true medical insurance also means removing the barriers to competition across state lines. If residents of Wyoming may purchase oranges from Florida, wine from France and mutual funds from Tokyo, why can't any and all Americans buy insurance (which is after all a *financial* product, not even a medical product or service) from outside of their state? For that matter, why can't they buy it from outside the country if the financial indemnity provided by a multinational institution serves their need for security in the event of health catastrophe? Most state-level insurance regulation should be declared unconstitutional and/or repealed on the grounds of undue interference with interstate commerce and individual liberty. A New Yorker shouldn't have to contemplate moving across the street to Connecticut just because state mandates have made health insurance four times more expensive in the state of New York, for the same consumer.

Level the playing field, because World War II is over and we thought we won

If employers get a tax break for providing health insurance, then individuals who purchase coverage directly from the insurance company should get the same break too. There is no moral or economic justification for preferences, privileges or prejudices to be tolerated in the tax code.

We are suffering to this day from the legacy of World War II-era price controls. In the 1940's companies were not permitted to raise wages to attract workers (now where's a good law like that when you need one?), but they were able to offer non-wage benefits, like pre-paid health plans, to get around the price control laws and make work more attractive than at the competitor's factory. The IRS gave its blessing to this scheme on October 26, 1943. Physician and author William C Waters M.D. calls this the first day of '*2 Days That Ruined Your Healthcare*'. WWII ended and with it the wage and price controls, but tax-privileged employer-provided health insurance endures to the present day and is the primary cause of the economic imbalance in this sector.

Loosening the coupling between employment and health insurance would also relieve the trauma of unemployment, because workers wouldn't necessarily have to lose their health insurance just because they lose their jobs – a double-whammy.

Give the money to the patients.

Whatever financial assistance the federal government allocates to health care should be in the form of block grants to the states for them to do with as they see fit, with the understanding that there will be no bailouts for irresponsible states at the expense of prudently-managed ones. Better yet would be to cut federal taxes so that states don't have to beg for money that never should have gone to Washington D.C. in the first place.

Whatever financial support states give toward health care should go directly to individual citizens so they can make their own decisions as to what policy to purchase (or not), what physician or other provider to seek for services.

Nobody ever spent other people's money as wisely as they spend their own. Health care cost inflation will be tamed the minute patients have the ability to negotiate with providers with the resources under their own command. As it is, only 13% of health care dollars spent in America are under the direct control of patients.

For the vast majority of Americans, it's not necessary to give them anything other than the freedom to do as they see fit with what is theirs. As a matter of policy, this means liberalizing policies in favor of Medical Savings Accounts (MSAs), and permitting association plans and other tax advantages for individuals and small-business owners, as is already allowed for large employers. When health insurance premiums can be paid in tax-free dollars, more people will have the means to be insured.

Tax deductions or credits for medical expenses and health insurance premiums (through any channel: individual, employer or other group) will result in more people getting insured.

70

Cut out the Legal Casino Mafia Middleman

Physicians in the U.S.A. collectively spend tens of billions of dollars each year defending themselves against malpractice lawsuits, 90% of which are eventually found to be frivolous as demonstrated by verdicts, but which cost $100,000 apiece to fight. As a result, physicians make decisions about tests and treatment increasingly on the basis of avoiding lawsuits as much or more than in the genuine best interest of the patient. Defensive medicine – unnecessary tests and procedures – wastes money, contributing to the health care cost inflation problem.

States like Texas have shown how the damage may be mitigated. By putting a cap of $250,000 on non-economic damages in 2003, Texas reduced the number of cases by over 80% and the number of physicians attracted to practice in the state increased 18% in four years.

Implementing 'loser-pays' laws, in which any plaintiff filing a claim found to be baseless must pay the legal costs of the defendant, would bring restraint to this out-of-control arena of legalized extortion.

Don't subsidize unhealthy products

Two of America's most serious health problems are obesity and smoking. This is not the fault of the health care system, but of individual habits and responsibility. Even so, government policy contributes to the problem by subsidizing certain products that contribute to bad health, like sugar, corn syrup and even tobacco ($1.3 billion in support from 1995 to 2011). This makes them cheaper to the consumer and more profitable to the producer than they would be under a free market, at the same time that the government is actively campaigning to dissuade the public from consuming them. Duh. This is just one more example of how special-interest-driven government interference works at cross-purposes to the general welfare.

Let this Patient Die

Some people want to 'reform' Obamacare, not repeal it. Now that we know what's in it, can't we remove what we don't like and keep the good parts?

A plan so deeply rooted in misperception, centralized planning, misinformation, mono-partisanship and political bullying, passed in the Senate in the wee hours of Christmas Eve 2009, is not salvageable. Medicare and RomneyCare at least had the virtue of being bipartisan efforts. But Obamacare was passed without a single Republican vote. 83% of physicians in the U.S. are opposed to it, to the point of retreating from their practices, opting out of Medicare, decreasing office hours or even quitting while they are ahead. The general public began to have buyer's remorse almost immediately after passage, and that sentiment has only grown stronger since. As of the end of 2012, 54% of Americans were opposed to universal coverage, the idea that it is the government's job to ensure that all Americans have healthcare coverage. The law is so unpopular that the department of Health and Human Services (HHS) withheld publishing its rules for how states and doctors will be required to comply with the law (13,000 pages and counting) until after the 2012 election was safely over. If the law is so warm and fuzzy, why did Louisiana and other states have to file a Freedom of Information Act request just to 'find out what's in it'? Former supporters of the bill are openly expressing astonishment at the destruction they see happening around them, like the physician who writes "Medicare made the rules and now punishes doctors for following them".

To fix what's wrong with medical care in America, we need REAL health insurance along with liberty, voluntary cooperation, free markets, the price system and the virtues of the free people of America. A true health insurance market thriving under free-market competition will provide the greatest range of choices possible to all of us, including today's uninsured. Such a market needs freedom and competition; not over-regulation, rationing and penalties; not a government takeover. Individuals, families and physicians should be the ones in charge; not the federal Department of Health and Human Services and committees that can't be recalled by voters.

74

The Hippocratic oath, taken by physicians for over two thousand years, pledges: "First, do no harm". America needs reform, but not just any reform. We cannot rush into top-down, government-directed economics out of an irresistible urge just to 'do something', convinced that "it can't possibly get any worse". It can always get worse. It *is* worse in almost every other country and is already getting worse here under Obamacare. Constructive reform has to be based on an accurate assessment of the circumstances and on sound economic principles.

Reversing Obamacare won't be easy this late in the game. The Administration and die-hard supporters of the law aren't standing down for a gentleman-general's winter camp; to the contrary, they are armed with virtually unlimited resources and mobilized to put down any trace of rebellion. The element of surprise won't be found in a frontal attack on an A.C.A. stronghold, like (metaphorically) George Washington's ambush of the Hessians at Trenton. It will come, rather, from all of the former and fair-weather supporters who never expected that the rising costs, rationing, shortages, loss of liberty, restriction of choices and deteriorating quality would fall so heavily upon them personally.

But reverse it we must, because living under this law's regime will be much dearer still than the cost of fighting it to the bitter end. The death panel rationing committee of the American citizenry has determined that this patient's life is not worth the cost of prolonging. It's time to pull the plug on Obamacare.

A word about charity

The existence and necessity of charity is not a failure; it is one of the great virtues of civilization, particularly the North American brand.

In political debates, the person who first invokes charity as part of the solution is often cast by the opponent as the automatic loser of the argument. "Aha! Your deficient solution leaves people starving and begging in the streets!" But not only is it appropriate to leave room for private, non-profit and/or religion-based local volunteer work, such work is essential to the health of the civil society. Citizens should not be led to believe that they are absolved of all responsibility once they have sent their tribute to Washington DC – or worse, that they have no responsibility because they don't earn enough to pay federal income taxes (more than 50% of American adults fit that category).

All reliable evidence demonstrates that the dollars spent and personal time donated voluntarily is far more effective than government programs that profess to accomplish similar goals. Again, people naturally spend their own money and time more carefully than they do other people's, and are more motivated by faith and by personal involvement, even when their motivation is the well-being of other people.

America has a great tradition of local, decentralized, diverse, mostly faith-based charity for poor relief, hospitals, educational endowments etc. That tradition is healthier and more dynamic in the United States than it is in Europe or any other nation on Earth. It is a treasure to be preserved and cultivated. Americans give more of their time and money than the citizens of any other nation, at any income level (not just the 'rich' who can 'afford it').

Yet by proposing a Washington DC-based solution to every real and imagined problem, 'progressive' politicians increasingly put the squeeze on private charity and local volunteerism. In vulgar marketing terms, government dollars crowd out private dollars and take market share away from the churches, foundations and volunteer organizations that traditionally did the work. This is not just economically inefficient; it is a moral hazard.

The volunteer who puts in time out of love for God or for his fellow man (or just because he wants to score points with that girl at the church social) does so on his/her own account, having personal involvement and connection to the people he or she is trying to help. Government bureaucrats who administer impersonal programs that crowd out charitable giving and volunteer work demand high salaries, ironclad job security and a host of other benefits procured by their collective bargaining unions, all at taxpayer expense, with next to zero personal connection to his or her 'clients'. This is a far cry from the great American tradition of giving.

All of the world's great religions – Christianity, Judaism, Islam, Hinduism, Shintoism, Buddhism, Zoroastrianism and more – reserve an indispensible place in human social life for private voluntary charity. But some activists behave as if they believe that all good comes from the state, only the state can do good, and little that does not come from the state could be good. That is how 'compassion' becomes defined as raising taxes on 'the rich', and anyone who opposes such policy is painted as an uncompassionate, heartless and greedy enemy of the 99%; the 'adamantly selfish'.

Even if you are not particularly religious (from Christmas- and Easter-only Christian to militant atheist), it should be possible for you to appreciate the value of private, voluntary charitable giving, and to recognize that pursuing policies that implicitly seek to suffocate it cannot possibly leave our society any healthier.

With this in mind, the place for charity work should be acknowledged and encouraged by the tax code and by legislated policy. The tax deductibility of charitable donations should be liberal, not assailed as 'loopholes'. Foundations should be given room to grow, not crowded out of the market. Physicians should be permitted to deduct services rendered free of charge from their taxable income. Legislative projects that seek to help the poor should not pretend to eradicate all poverty for all time – an impossibility – but to do what a prudent government can do while leaving the lion's share of the work to the people who do it best and at the lowest cost. Severely infringing upon the rights of 90% of the people by force in order to 'solve' the problems of the 10% is unwise and destructive.

Private, voluntary charity deserves at least an equal if not greater status in any health care reform than either government or business participation.

How?

Everything in this pamphlet so far has been about *why*: Why Obamacare is wrongheaded, destructive and doomed (or why we are doomed if we don't roll *It* back.) The question of *how*, that is, the strategy and tactics to bring about repeal and effective reform, is a whole other topic for political experts. But it boils down to one word: *Senate*.

The U.S. Senate is the primary obstacle to reform and therefore needs to be the focus of grassroots pressure.

The Supreme Court has punted[9], which is bad news but not fundamentally an obstacle. Republicans reside in a supermajority of state mansions, and thereby hold significant power (if they choose to exercise it) of frustrating the federal government's grand plans. The U.S. House of Representatives has voted dozens of

---

[9] In June 2012 the Supreme Court upheld the constitutionality of the individual mandate on the grounds of Congress' power to tax, in spite of the fact that the law does not say 'tax' and its supporters denied to the gods that the individual mandate was a tax while they were selling it.

times against provisions of the A.C.A. since it passed, including voting to scrap the whole thing in July 2012. These votes have been symbolic, of course, since it takes two to tango, and the dance partner has decided it prefers the goosestep. But public disenchantment will grow as people personally experience more and more of the destructive effects of the provisions of the law. That disenchantment must be energetically harnessed and directed at the chamber and members thereof that insist upon steamrolling over the wishes, liberty and prosperity of the people.

That's your job.

Don't take my word for it!

BIBLIOGRAPHY AND RESOURCES

I'm not making this stuff up. I couldn't make this stuff up. I am indebted to dozens of researchers whose pioneering work is the source of my facts and statistics. To verify the facts, get more in-depth information and connect with people and organizations who are committed to fighting for truth, justice and the American way, here are a few indispensible resources:

Official companion web page to this book:

- www.HHCapitalism.com/p/Obamacare.html
  Updated notes, facts, statistics and more.

Books:

- McCaughey, Betsy, PhD, <u>Beating Obamacare</u>, published by Regnery Publishing Inc 2013. Ms. McCaughey has been fighting against socialized medicine at least since HillaryCare in 1993.

- Pipes, Sally C, The Truth About Obamacare, pub. by Regnery Publishing Inc, 2010. Don't say no one warned you.

- Tate, Nick J. Obamacare Survival Guide: The Affordable Care Act and What It Means for You and Your Healthcare, pub. by Humanix Books, 2012.

- Pipes, Sally C, The Pipes Plan: The Top 10 Ways to Dismantle Obamacare, pub. by Regnery Publishing Inc, 2012.

- Turner, Capretta, Miller and Moffit, Why Obamacare is Wrong for America, pub. by HarperCollins, 2011.

- Waters M.D., William C., 2 Days That Ruined Your Healthcare, pub. by Logicon Press, 2008.

- Gratzer, David, Why Obama's Government Takeover of Health Care Will Be a Disaster, pub. by Encounter Books, 2009.

Organizations and Online Resources

- The Pacific Research Institute, Sally Pipes, President: http://pacificresearch.org

- Americans for Prosperity:
  http://americansforprosperity.org/issues/healthcare-entitlements
- The Cato Institute
  http://www.cato.org/research/health-care
- The Heritage Foundation:
  http://www.heritage.org/initiatives/health-care
- America's Medical Society, Dr. Adam Dorin M.D., Founder:
  http://americasmedicalsociety.com
- American Association of Physicians and Surgeons: http://www.aapsonline.org
- www.Docs4PatientCare.org
  "We are an organization of concerned physicians committed to the establishment of a health care system that preserves the sanctity of the doctor-patient relationship, promotes quality of care, supports affordable access to all Americans, and protects patients' freedom of choice."
- '121 Reasons to Reject Obama-Reid-PelosiCare', online article pub. November 2009 by Howard Hyde on www.HHCapitalism.com. Don't say *I* never warned you.

About the Author

HOWARD HYDE has no formal credentials whatsoever qualifying him to write this pamphlet. He is neither a doctor, nor a public official, nor a professor, nor a professional economist. He holds no certifications or licenses in Medicine, Economics or Public Policy. He doesn't have any advanced degrees, and the B.A. degree he does have is in Music (University of Southern California Thornton School, 1990).

For this reason the reader is cautioned not to believe anything herein contained on blind faith, but to check every fact, carefully analyze the logic of every argument and watch out for rhetorical slights of tongue and pen. Only by being vigilant, skeptical and critical can the citizen-voter prevent being misled by charlatans posing as experts.

www.ingramcontent.com/pod-product-compliance
Lightning Source LLC
Chambersburg PA
CBHW022123280326
41933CB00007B/520